# Iodine

## A Beginner's Quick Start Guide on Its Health Use Cases, With a Potential 3-Step Plan on How to Get Started

MARY GOLANNA

# Introduction

Most people know iodine as the substance that's added to salt to prevent goiter, a condition that causes the thyroid gland to enlarge and swell. However, iodine has many other benefits beyond just preventing goiter. In fact, iodine is an essential mineral that plays a crucial role in maintaining good health.

Did you know that iodine is necessary for the production of thyroid hormones? These hormones regulate metabolism, growth, and development in our bodies. Without enough iodine, our bodies can't produce enough thyroid hormones, leading to hypothyroidism, a condition that causes fatigue, weight gain, and depression.

But that's not all. Iodine also plays a vital role in brain development, particularly during pregnancy and infancy. It helps ensure that the brain develops properly and can affect cognitive function throughout life. Iodine also has anti-inflammatory properties and can help protect against certain types of cancers, such as breast and prostate cancer.

Now that you know how important iodine is for your health, you may be wondering how to ensure you're getting enough of it. The good news is that iodine is found in a variety of foods, including seafood, seaweed, dairy products, and eggs. However, some people may need to supplement with iodine, especially if they have an iodine deficiency or are pregnant.

In this guide, we'll explore everything you need to know about the following;

- What is Iodine?
- How does Iodine work?
- Benefits of Iodine and Two Main Forms of Iodine
- Symptoms, Causes, and Treatment of Iodine Deficiency
- Use Cases, Pros, and Cons
- Recommended Dosage and Usage
- Potential Side Effects
- Step Plan To Get Started with Iodine
- Safety Precautions and Considerations
- Food Sources and How Diet can play a role in getting enough Iodine

By the end of this post, you'll have a better understanding of why iodine is so important for your health and how to ensure you're getting enough of it.

# Table of Contents

# CHAPTER 1: WHAT IS IODINE

Iodine is a chemical element with the symbol I and atomic number 53. It is a halogen, and like other halogens, it is found in the periodic table in group 17. Iodine is a relatively rare element in the Earth's crust, but it is essential for human health.

The thyroid gland uses iodine to produce two hormones: thyroxine (T4) and triiodothyronine (T3). These hormones are involved in regulating various metabolic processes, including energy production, protein synthesis, and the growth and development of organs and tissues. Without adequate levels of iodine, the thyroid gland cannot produce enough thyroid hormone, leading to a range of health issues.

The discovery of this element is attributed to a chemist who accidentally found it while trying to extract a different substance from seaweed ash. He noticed purple vapors and realized that a new element was present. This element was given a name derived from a Greek word meaning violet-colored.

Today, this element is primarily obtained from natural sources such as seafood and seaweed, as well as through fortified foods. It is essential for maintaining healthy thyroid function and preventing hypothyroidism, making it an important element for human health.

## How does Iodine Work?

Iodine works in the body by regulating the production of thyroid hormones, which are essential for proper metabolism and growth. The thyroid gland absorbs iodine from the blood and uses it to produce two important hormones: thyroxine (T4) and triiodothyronine (T3). These hormones are involved in regulating a wide range of metabolic processes throughout the body, including energy production, protein synthesis, and the growth and development of organs and tissues.

When there is adequate iodine in the diet, the thyroid gland can produce enough of these hormones to maintain normal bodily functions. But if iodine levels are too low, the thyroid gland must work harder to try to produce enough thyroid hormones, leading to enlargement of the gland known as goiter. If iodine deficiency persists, however, the thyroid gland may eventually become unable to produce sufficient thyroid hormones, leading to hypothyroidism.

Iodine also has antimicrobial properties and can help prevent infections. It may do this by interfering with the ability of bacteria and viruses to reproduce and spread. Additionally, research has suggested that iodine may have anti-cancer effects, although more studies are needed to fully understand this aspect of its functioning in the body.

Overall, iodine is a crucial nutrient that plays an essential role in maintaining optimal health and functioning. Without enough iodine in the diet, the body cannot produce enough thyroid hormones, leading to a range of health issues and impairments.

## Benefits of Iodine

Iodine is necessary for the production of vital hormones and helps promote proper growth and development. But there are many other benefits to getting enough iodine in your diet. Here are just a few:

### Healthy thyroid function

The thyroid gland requires iodine to produce thyroid hormones, which regulate various bodily functions such as metabolism, growth, and development. Iodine deficiency can lead to an enlarged thyroid gland (goiter) and hypothyroidism, which can cause fatigue, weight gain, and other health issues. By maintaining adequate levels of iodine, the thyroid gland can function properly, helping to ensure overall health.

### Brain development

Iodine plays a crucial role in fetal and infant brain development. Adequate iodine intake during pregnancy and early childhood can help ensure proper brain development, leading to better cognitive function throughout life. This vital nutrient helps the brain develop its complex network of neural connections, promoting healthy brain function.

A lack of iodine during the critical stages of brain development can result in cognitive delays and lower IQ. Recent studies have shown that iodine supplementation in pregnant women can significantly improve cognitive outcomes for their children. Furthermore, countries with iodine fortification programs have seen significant improvements in cognitive function among their populations.

### Protection against certain cancers

However, recent studies have shown that iodine can also protect against certain types of cancer, specifically thyroid and breast cancer. This is due to its antioxidant and anti-inflammatory properties that help prevent cellular damage and mutations in DNA that can lead to cancer formation.

Evidence suggests that iodine can inhibit tumor growth and induce apoptosis (programmed cell death) in cancer cells. Additionally, iodine has been found to block the effects of estrogen, which is a hormone that can promote breast cancer development. Therefore, incorporating iodine-rich foods in the diet, such as seaweed, fish, and dairy products, may be beneficial in reducing the risk of cancer.

### Immune system support

Iodine offers valuable immune system support owing to its antimicrobial properties. These properties make it challenging for viruses and bacteria to reproduce and propagate within the body. Iodine also promotes an acidic environment in the body, which further impairs the survival of pathogens.

A growing body of evidence shows that iodine supplementation can be useful in preventing infectious respiratory illnesses such as the cold and flu. By strengthening the immune system, iodine bolsters the body's natural defenses against the spread of these viruses and bacteria, contributing to better overall health and well-being.

## Improved energy levels

Iodine is a crucial mineral that plays a significant role in ensuring optimal health and well-being. One of the main benefits of iodine is its positive impact on energy levels. The mineral helps regulate the thyroid gland, which is responsible for controlling metabolism in the body.

When the thyroid is functioning normally, iodine helps to improve the production and utilization of energy, thereby leading to increased physical performance and higher energy levels. This makes iodine intake vital for athletes, individuals experiencing fatigue or chronic tiredness, and those who want to boost their overall energy levels and productivity.

## Improved metabolism

Iodine is an essential nutrient that plays a crucial role in regulating metabolism. Research suggests that adequate iodine levels can promote healthy thyroid function, which, in turn, can lead to more efficient calorie burning and better weight management.

When there is a deficiency of iodine in the body, the thyroid gland works harder to produce essential hormones, slowing down metabolism and leading to weight gain. Incorporating sources of iodine into the diet can, therefore, boost metabolism and promote a healthy weight.

**Improved heart health**

Iodine is a crucial mineral for regulating blood pressure, preventing atherosclerosis, reducing the risk of hypertension and other heart-related conditions, and consequently promoting better overall cardiovascular health. It achieves this by controlling the production of hormones crucial to heart function, such as thyroid hormones.

In addition, adequate iodine intake also promotes the proper functioning of the endothelial cells, which line the arteries and regulate blood flow. Research indicates that individuals who have insufficient iodine intake have an increased likelihood of developing cardiovascular disease, underscoring the importance of incorporating iodine-rich foods into one's diet.

By getting enough iodine in your diet, you can ensure that your thyroid gland functions properly and maintain overall health. Adequate intake of this essential mineral provides numerous benefits and helps to support a range of bodily processes. Additionally, iodine is necessary for proper brain development and function, which is especially important during pregnancy and early childhood.

**Two Main Forms of Iodine**

While iodine is found in various forms in nature, two main forms of iodine are consumed by humans:

## Inorganic iodine

This type of iodine is found in nature and is commonly used in the manufacturing of industrial products such as dyes, disinfectants, and photographic film. Inorganic iodine can also be found in some types of seaweed and seafood. While it is important for various industrial processes, inorganic iodine is not typically consumed by humans due to its potential toxicity at high levels.

## Organic iodine

Organic iodine occurs naturally in the environment and is found in some foods such as dairy, eggs, and seafood. It is also added to some dietary supplements, particularly those marketed as iodine sources for vegans or vegetarians.

Organic iodine is an essential nutrient for human health, as it is necessary for the production of thyroid hormones, which regulate metabolism, growth, and development. Unlike inorganic iodine, organic iodine is safe for human consumption when taken in recommended doses.

In contrast, inorganic iodine is primarily used in industrial applications and is not intended for human consumption due to its potential toxicity. Overall, understanding the differences between these two forms of iodine is important for ensuring optimal health and well-being.

## Various Forms of Iodine

There are several forms of iodine available, each with its own unique properties and uses. Here are some of the most common forms of iodine:

## Potassium iodide

Potassium iodide is a salt of iodine that is commonly used in medicine and other applications. It is often used as a supplement to prevent iodine deficiency, particularly in areas where soil and food sources are low in iodine. Potassium iodide is also used in the treatment of thyroid problems, including goiter and hyperthyroidism.

Additionally, it is used as a radiation protection in nuclear emergencies, as it can help protect the thyroid gland from radioactive iodine. Potassium iodide is generally safe when used as directed, although excessive intake can lead to side effects such as nausea, vomiting, and abdominal pain. It's important to speak with a healthcare provider before taking potassium iodide supplements to ensure that they're safe and effective for your needs.

## Iodine tincture

Iodine tincture is a versatile liquid form of iodine that is commonly used to disinfect wounds and surgical sites. It is a skin antiseptic that is applied prior to surgery to reduce the risk of infection. In addition, it can also be used to treat skin infections caused by bacteria and fungi. The solution works by penetrating the cell wall of microbes, thereby destroying them.

Furthermore, iodine tincture is a powerful disinfectant that can effectively kill a wide range of microorganisms, including bacteria, viruses, and spores. Due to its broad-spectrum activity and ease of use, it is a popular antiseptic choice in healthcare settings.

## Lugol's solution

Iodine, a chemical element found in the periodic table, is utilized in the medical sector as Lugol's Solution - a potent combination of potassium iodide and elemental iodine. This solution is widely used as a disinfectant, to cure iodine deficiency, and is most commonly utilized to prepare the thyroid gland for surgical procedures.

Its effectiveness lies in the antibacterial properties of iodine. The solution kills bacteria by penetrating their cell wall and disrupting their metabolic pathways. In addition, it regulates the thyroid gland by supplying it with the amount of iodine it requires, thereby preventing thyroid diseases.

## Radioactive iodine

Radioactive iodine is a powerful diagnostic and treatment tool for hyperthyroidism and thyroid cancer. When given orally, it selectively targets the thyroid gland, destroying cells and reducing the size of the gland.

Its effectiveness is due to the fact that the thyroid is one of the few organs that will absorb iodine, making this form of iodine highly effective for treating these conditions. Despite its powerful capabilities, radioactive iodine must be used with caution due to its potentially harmful effects on healthy cells.

## Povidone-iodine

Povidone-iodine is a chemical complex of iodine that is commonly used as an antiseptic in medical and surgical settings. It works by releasing iodine slowly, which kills or prevents the growth of bacteria, viruses, and fungi. Povidone-iodine is used for skin disinfection prior to surgery, as well as for wound care and treatment of infections such as impetigo.

It is also used in dental procedures and to disinfect medical equipment. Povidone-iodine is generally safe when used as directed, although some people may experience skin irritation or allergic reactions. It's important to speak with a healthcare provider before using povidone-iodine, particularly if you have a history of iodine allergy or thyroid problems.

## Organic iodine compounds

Organic iodine compounds are utilized as contrast agents in medical imaging procedures due to their ability to provide better visualization of bodily structures. These compounds contain iodine molecules that are bound to organic molecules, providing a stable and safe delivery of the element Iodine.

This allows for improved imaging of various organs, including the brain, liver, and kidneys. Additionally, organic iodine compounds are preferred over non-organic compounds due to their lower toxicity and reduced risk of adverse reactions.

Overall, iodine is an essential nutrient that plays a vital role in thyroid function and overall health. While there are various forms of iodine available, it's important to use them under medical supervision and in moderation to avoid negative health effects.

# CHAPTER 2: USE CASES

Iodine is important for many aspects of human health, and there are several health problems that can be treated or prevented by ensuring adequate iodine intake. Here are some examples:

## Hypothyroidism

Iodine is an essential mineral that plays a crucial role in maintaining a healthy thyroid gland. The thyroid gland produces hormones that regulate metabolism and energy levels in the body. If you're not getting enough iodine in your diet, it can lead to an underactive thyroid gland (hypothyroidism).

Supplementing with iodine can help alleviate symptoms like fatigue, weight gain, and sluggishness. However, it's important to note that excessive iodine intake can also be harmful, so it's important to get the right amount of iodine for your body's needs.

## Goiter

A goiter is an enlargement of the thyroid gland, often caused by iodine deficiency. Taking iodine supplements can help shrink the goiter and prevent it from growing larger. In addition to supplementing with iodine, it's also important to eat a well-balanced diet that includes foods rich in iodine, such as seafood, dairy products, and eggs. If you suspect that you have a goiter, it's important to see a healthcare provider to determine the cause and appropriate treatment.

## Fibrocystic Breast Disease

Fibrocystic breast disease is a common condition characterized by painful lumps in the breasts. Iodine supplementation has been found to help alleviate symptoms of fibrocystic breast disease. Studies have shown that iodine supplementation can reduce breast pain and tenderness, as well as the size and number of breast cysts. However, more research is needed to fully understand how iodine affects breast health.

## Radiation Exposure

Potassium iodide (KI) is a form of iodine that can be used to protect against radiation exposure. KI works by saturating the thyroid gland with iodine, which prevents it from absorbing radioactive iodine that may be released during a nuclear disaster. It's important to note that KI should only be taken under the guidance of a healthcare provider in the event of a radiation emergency.

## Breast Cancer

Studies have shown that iodine may play a role in preventing breast cancer. Iodine has been found to induce apoptosis (cell death) in breast cancer cells, and researchers believe that low iodine levels may be a risk factor for developing the disease.

However, more research is needed to fully understand the relationship between iodine and breast cancer.

## Thyroid Cancer

Iodine may also be effective in treating thyroid cancer. Radioactive iodine therapy is a common treatment option for thyroid cancer, as the thyroid gland absorbs iodine more readily than other tissues.

This allows the radioactive iodine to target and destroy cancerous thyroid cells. However, not all types of thyroid cancer respond to this treatment, so it's important to discuss your options with a healthcare provider.

## Skin Health

Iodine may also be beneficial for skin health. Topical iodine solutions have been used to treat skin conditions like warts, psoriasis, and eczema. Iodine can also help improve skin hydration and elasticity, which can reduce the appearance of fine lines and wrinkles.

However, it's important to note that excessive iodine intake can also lead to skin irritation and other adverse effects, so it's important to consult with a healthcare provider before using iodine for skin health purposes

## Iodine Deficiency

Lack of iodine can lead to a condition known as iodine deficiency. Iodine deficiency is a major global health problem, affecting an estimated 2 billion people worldwide. It is most common in areas with little access to iodine-rich foods and iodized salt. Symptoms of severe iodine deficiency can include:

## Enlarged thyroid gland (goiter)

An enlarged thyroid gland, also known as goiter, is a common symptom of iodine deficiency. When the body doesn't get enough iodine, the thyroid gland cannot produce enough thyroid hormone, leading to an enlarged gland.

This swelling can cause discomfort and pain in the neck, as well as difficulty swallowing or breathing. In addition, an enlarged thyroid gland can be unsightly and impact a person's self-esteem. To prevent the development of goiter, it's important to consume iodine-rich foods or take iodine supplements.

## Fatigue

Iodine plays a crucial role in the production of energy within the body. Hence, when there is an iodine deficiency, it can lead to a persistent feeling of fatigue and weakness. This occurs due to a reduction in the amount of thyroid hormones produced, which are responsible for regulating metabolism and energy expenditure. The energy deficit experienced by individuals with an iodine deficiency can manifest in various ways, including lethargy, weakness, and a decreased ability to concentrate.

## Weight gain

Low levels of iodine have a direct impact on metabolism, which in turn affects weight gain. This deficiency leads to a slower metabolism, making it difficult for the body to burn calories and lose weight.

Additionally, the body is forced to store excess calories, causing significant weight gain over time. This can lead to various complications, including obesity, diabetes, and other metabolic disorders. Adequate iodine intake can help regulate metabolism and maintain a healthy weight, making it essential to consume enough iodine-rich foods.

## Mental fog

Iodine plays a crucial role in brain function, and its deficiency can lead to numerous cognitive impairments. One of the most common symptoms of iodine deficiency is difficulty concentrating and memory problems.

This happens because iodine is essential for the production of thyroid hormones, which regulate brain metabolism, and a deficiency can lead to decreased activity in various parts of the brain. Besides, iodine deficiency can also cause developmental delays, depression, and other neurological disorders.

## Developmental Delays and intellectual disabilities in Children

Iodine deficiency is a serious concern for pregnant women and young children as it can result in developmental delays and intellectual disabilities. The developmental effects of iodine deficiency are significant with children experiencing stunted growth, cognitive impairment, and reduced school performance.

In addition, iodine deficiency during pregnancy can increase the risk of stillbirth, miscarriage, and premature delivery. These adverse outcomes can be prevented with adequate iodine intake through a balanced diet or supplements. It is essential for healthcare providers to educate and guide pregnant women and parents on the importance of iodine for the proper growth and development of their children.

## Dry skin and hair

Dry skin and hair are common symptoms of iodine deficiency. The lack of iodine in the body can lead to a decrease in the production of hormones that play a crucial role in maintaining healthy skin and hair. This deficiency leads to reduced oil production in the skin, which makes it dry and prone to itchiness, cracking, and peeling.

It can also lower the quality of hair, making it brittle, dull, and prone to breakage. If left untreated, the condition can become severe, leading to other health complications. Therefore, it is crucial to consume iodine-rich foods or supplements to maintain healthy skin and hair.

It's important to note that these symptoms can also be caused by other health conditions, so it's essential to speak with a healthcare provider if you're experiencing any of these symptoms to determine the underlying cause.

## Causes of Iodine Deficiency

There are several causes of iodine deficiency, including:

1. **Inadequate intake:** One of the most common causes of iodine deficiency is simply not consuming enough iodine in the diet. This can occur if a person does not consume enough iodine-rich foods or if they live in an area with low levels of iodine in the soil.

2. **Soil depletion:** The amount of iodine present in soil can vary depending on the region and can affect the amount of iodine present in food grown in that soil. In areas where the soil is depleted of iodine, the plants and animals raised in that region will also have lower levels of iodine.

3. **Vegetarian or vegan diets:** People who follow vegetarian or vegan diets may be at higher risk for iodine deficiency since many plant-based foods are not good sources of iodine.

4. **Pregnancy and breastfeeding:** Pregnant and breastfeeding women require more iodine to support the healthy development of their babies. If they don't get enough iodine through their diet, they may become deficient.

5. **Goitrogenic foods:** Consuming excessive amounts of goitrogenic foods, such as soy products and cruciferous vegetables like broccoli and cauliflower, can interfere with iodine absorption and contribute to iodine deficiency.

It's important to note that some countries have implemented mandatory salt iodization programs to address iodine deficiency. If you're concerned about your iodine intake, speak with a healthcare provider or registered dietitian to determine the best course of action.

## Treatment For Iodine Deficiency

The treatment for iodine deficiency depends on the severity of the deficiency and the underlying cause. Here are some common approaches to treating iodine deficiency:

- Increase iodine intake through diet: Consuming more iodine-rich foods can help increase iodine levels in the body. Foods that are high in iodine include seafood, seaweed, eggs, and dairy products.
- Use iodized salt: Iodized salt is a common way to ensure adequate iodine intake, as it's widely available and easy to add to meals.
- Iodine supplements: Iodine supplements can be prescribed to people with moderate to severe iodine deficiency. It's important to speak with a healthcare provider before taking any supplements, as excessive iodine intake can be harmful.
- Treat underlying conditions: If an underlying condition is causing the iodine deficiency, such as an autoimmune disorder or gastrointestinal disorder, it may be necessary to treat that condition to improve iodine absorption.
- Monitor thyroid function: People with iodine deficiency should have their thyroid function monitored regularly to evaluate the effectiveness of treatment and ensure that there are no complications.

It's important to note that while iodine deficiency can have negative health effects, excessive iodine intake can also be harmful. Speak with a healthcare provider or registered dietitian to determine the best course of action for your specific needs.

# CHAPTER 3: PROS AND CONS

In this chapter, we will explore some of the pros and cons of iodine, including its essential role as a nutrient, medical applications, and potential risks associated with excessive intake or environmental concerns. Understanding the various aspects of iodine can help individuals make informed decisions about their diet, supplement use, and overall health.

**Advantages of Iodine**

The following are some of the most notable advantages of iodine:

**1. Versatile:**

Iodine is a versatile nutrient that can be consumed in various forms, including supplements, iodized salt, and food sources. This makes it easy to incorporate into your daily routine and ensures that you're getting adequate levels of iodine. Whether you prefer seafood, dairy products, or supplements, there are multiple options to suit your needs.

**2. Effective:**

Iodine is an essential nutrient that plays a crucial role in thyroid function and overall health. Adequate iodine intake can help support healthy brain development, boost the immune system, and reduce the risk of certain cancers. By incorporating more iodine-rich foods into your diet and speaking with a healthcare provider, you can help ensure that you're getting adequate levels of this important nutrient.

### 3.  Widely available:

Iodine is widely available, making it accessible to people around the world. Many countries have implemented iodine supplementation programs to address deficiencies and improve public health. Whether you live in a developed or developing country, you can likely find iodine-rich foods, supplements, or iodized salt to meet your needs.

### 4.  Safe:

Iodine is generally safe when consumed in appropriate amounts, and toxicity is rare. However, it's important to speak with a healthcare provider before taking iodine supplements, as excessive intake can be harmful. With proper guidance and supervision, iodine can be safely incorporated into your diet to support overall health and well-being.

### 5.  Affordable:

Iodine-rich foods, such as seafood, eggs, and dairy products, are widely available and affordable. Iodized salt is also inexpensive and readily available in most regions. This makes it easy for people from all economic backgrounds to incorporate iodine into their diets without breaking the bank. Additionally, supplements can be affordable and may be covered by insurance in some cases.

Overall, the advantages of using iodine are numerous and include versatility, effectiveness, availability, safety, and affordability. By incorporating more iodine-rich foods into your diet and speaking with a healthcare provider, you can help ensure that you're getting adequate levels of this essential nutrient to support your overall health and well-being.

## Disadvantages of Iodine

The following are some potential disadvantages associated with iodine:

### 1.  Potential toxicity

Excessive intake of iodine in the form of potassium iodide can lead to potentially harmful effects on the human body. The thyroid gland is particularly sensitive to excess iodine, which can lead to thyroid dysfunction and a range of other health complications.

It is crucial to monitor iodine intake carefully, especially in regions where there is a high concentration of iodine in the soil or water supply. Overconsumption of iodine can have severe consequences and pose a significant risk to human health.

### 2.  Allergic reactions

Allergic reactions can pose a serious threat to individuals exposed to iodine. It is essential to note that some people are particularly allergic to iodine, and the resulting allergic reactions can be quite severe. Symptoms of an allergic reaction may include itching, hives, swelling, and difficulty breathing.

In severe allergic reactions, anaphylaxis may present itself, which can lead to shock, loss of consciousness, and even death. Therefore, it is imperative to take extra precautions when using iodine-containing products or undergoing any medical procedures involving iodine. If someone suspects they might be allergic, seeking medical advice before exposure is essential to avoid risk and ensure safety.

### 3.  Interference with medication

When consumed in excessive amounts, iodine can have an adverse effect on medication absorption, potentially reducing its effectiveness. Lithium, a medication used to treat bipolar disorder, is one such drug that may be affected.

Antibiotics such as tetracyclines and quinolones can also have their effectiveness reduced when taken in conjunction with high levels of iodine. It's important for individuals to monitor their iodine intake and speak with their healthcare provider to ensure optimal medication absorption.

### 4.  Environmental concerns

Excess iodine in the environment can lead to negative impacts on aquatic life and other ecosystems. Iodine can accumulate in soil and water, leading to toxic levels that can harm marine organisms, disrupt food chains, and subsequently degrade ecosystems. Similarly, elevated levels of iodine in agricultural soils can lead to reduced crop yield and quality, thereby damaging the agricultural sector.

Moreover, excess iodine in drinking water has been linked to various health risks, including thyroid dysfunction and an increased risk of cancer. Thus, it is crucial to regulate iodine levels in the environment to protect various ecosystems and minimize the risk to human health.

Overall, while iodine is an important nutrient, it is important to be mindful of potential risks associated with both inadequate and excessive iodine intake. As with any supplement or medication, it is always best to consult with a healthcare professional before making any changes to your iodine intake.

# CHAPTER 4:
# RECOMMENDED DOSAGE AND USAGE

Excessive iodine intake can lead to health problems such as thyroid dysfunction, so it's important to be mindful of dosage and usage when taking supplements or consuming iodine-rich foods. The upper limit for iodine intake is 1,100 micrograms per day for adults, which should not be exceeded without medical supervision.

While iodine is an essential nutrient, it's generally best to aim for adequate intake through a balanced diet rather than relying on supplements. However, if you are concerned about your iodine intake or have been advised by a healthcare provider to take an iodine supplement, it's important to follow the recommended dosage and usage instructions carefully.

Avoid taking too much iodine, as this can interfere with thyroid function and lead to health problems. It's always best to consult with a healthcare provider to determine the appropriate dosage for your individual needs.

**Potential Side Effects**

Although iodine is an essential nutrient, excessive intake can lead to health problems such as thyroid dysfunction. Some potential side effects of too much iodine include:

## 1.  Thyroid dysfunction:

The thyroid gland is responsible for producing hormones that regulate metabolism and other bodily functions. Excessive iodine intake can cause the thyroid gland to become overactive (hyperthyroidism) or underactive (hypothyroidism), leading to a range of symptoms such as weight changes, fatigue, and mood swings. It's important to maintain a balance of iodine intake to avoid these negative effects on the thyroid gland.

## 2.  Digestive issues:

High doses of iodine can be irritating to the digestive tract and can cause nausea, vomiting, and diarrhea. It's important to follow the recommended daily intake of iodine to avoid these unpleasant digestive symptoms.

## 3.  Metallic taste:

Consuming high doses of iodine can cause a metallic taste in the mouth. This is usually a temporary symptom that resolves once iodine intake is reduced.

## 4.  Acne:

Some people may experience acne breakouts when consuming high doses of iodine. This is thought to be due to the way iodine interacts with the skin's oil glands. Reducing iodine intake can help alleviate these symptoms.

## 5.  Thyroid cancer:

While iodine deficiency has been linked to an increased risk of thyroid cancer, some studies have suggested that excessive iodine intake may also increase the risk of certain types of thyroid cancer. However, more research is needed to fully understand the relationship between iodine intake and thyroid cancer.

It's important to note that most people do not experience any adverse side effects from consuming iodine in moderate amounts through diet or supplements. However, if you have any concerns about your iodine intake or are experiencing any unusual symptoms, it's important to speak with a healthcare provider. They can help determine whether any changes to your iodine intake or other treatments may be necessary.

# CHAPTER 5: 3-STEP PLAN TO GET STARTED WITH IODINE

If you are considering increasing your iodine intake, it is important to know the recommended daily amount and follow a healthy 3-step plan to get started.

- **Step 1: Consult a healthcare professional**

It is important to always consult a healthcare provider before making any changes to your iodine intake, as excessive iodine can lead to health problems such as thyroid dysfunction. A doctor or other medical professional can help determine the appropriate dosage for your individual needs, taking into account any underlying health conditions and other medication you are taking. Additionally, they can provide valuable information on any potential side effects or interactions between iodine and other supplements or medications.

- **Step 2: Start slow and gradually increase your intake**

It is best to start slowly with any dietary change, including iodine intake. Begin with the daily recommended amount or slightly below it and gradually increase over time if necessary. If you are taking a supplement, be sure to follow the dosage instructions carefully and do not exceed the upper limit of 1,100 micrograms per day for adults without medical supervision.

- **Step 3: Monitor your health and adjust accordingly**

Once you begin taking an iodine supplement or consuming more iodine-rich foods, it is important to monitor your health and adjust your intake as needed. If you experience any adverse side effects such as digestive issues, skin reactions, or thyroid dysfunction, speak with a healthcare provider as soon as possible. They can help you determine the appropriate course of action and provide any necessary medical treatment.

By following this 3-step plan, you can get started with iodine and ensure that your body has the essential nutrients it needs to function properly. Remember to consult a healthcare professional before making any major changes to your diet or taking supplements.

# CHAPTER 6: SAFETY PRECAUTIONS AND CONSIDERATIONS

When taking iodine, it is important to follow the recommended dose and safety precautions to avoid side effects or adverse reactions. Here are some safety precautions and considerations to keep in mind:

- Consult with your healthcare provider before taking any iodine supplements or medication.
- Avoid taking large doses of iodine as it can cause serious side effects such as nausea, vomiting, diarrhea, thyroid problems, and even coma.
- If you have a thyroid condition, such as an overactive or underactive thyroid, speak with your doctor to determine if iodine supplementation is safe for you.
- Pregnant and breastfeeding women should not take iodine supplements without consulting their healthcare provider first.
- Do not mix iodine supplements with other medications without consulting a healthcare professional as it may cause dangerous interactions.
- Always take iodine supplements with a full glass of water to avoid irritation to the stomach lining.

- Store iodine supplements in a cool, dry place away from direct sunlight.
- If you experience any adverse reactions, such as skin rash, joint pain, or swelling, stop taking iodine immediately, and seek medical attention.

Following these safety precautions and considerations will help you ensure that taking iodine is safe and effective for your needs.

### Who can Take Iodine?

Here are the different categories of people who can benefit from taking iodine supplements and their descriptions:

1. **Individuals with Iodine Deficiency**:

People living in areas where the soil is deficient in iodine or those who do not consume enough iodine-rich foods may benefit from iodine supplements. Iodine is essential for thyroid function, and a deficiency can lead to an enlarged thyroid gland (goiter), hypothyroidism, and intellectual disability.

2. **Pregnant and Breastfeeding Women**:

Pregnant and breastfeeding women require higher amounts of iodine to support fetal and infant development. Studies suggest that iodine supplementation during pregnancy can improve cognitive function in children.

3. **People with Thyroid Problems**:

Individuals with thyroid problems such as hyperthyroidism or hypothyroidism may benefit from iodine supplementation. However, iodine supplementation should only be done under the guidance of a healthcare provider as it can worsen certain thyroid conditions.

## 4.  People Undergoing Radiation Treatment:

People undergoing radiation treatment, particularly for head and neck cancer, may benefit from iodine supplementation to protect the thyroid gland from the harmful effects of radiation.

## 5.  Vegans and Vegetarians:

Vegans and vegetarians may not consume enough iodine-rich foods such as seaweed, seafood, and dairy products. Therefore, they may benefit from iodine supplementation.

It's important to note that while iodine supplementation is generally safe, excessive intake can lead to adverse effects. It's crucial to speak with a healthcare provider before taking any supplement to determine appropriate dosing and ensure it is right for your specific health needs and condition.

# CHAPTER 7: FOOD SOURCES OF IODINE

In addition to supplementation, you can get iodine from natural sources.

Here are some of the best iodine-rich foods:

1. **Seafood:**

Seafood is one of the best sources of iodine, particularly seaweed. One gram of seaweed can contain up to 2000 micrograms of iodine. Other types of seafood such as shrimp, tuna, and cod are also good sources of iodine.

2. **Dairy Products:**

Dairy products such as milk, cheese, and yogurt are good sources of iodine. A cup of milk contains about 56 micrograms of iodine, while a cup of plain yogurt can contain up to 90 micrograms of iodine.

3. **Eggs:**

Eggs are a good source of iodine, with one large egg containing about 24 micrograms of iodine. The amount of odine in eggs can vary depending on the hens' diet and other factors.

4. **Iodized Salt:**

Iodized salt is a common source of iodine and is added to many processed foods. One gram of iodized salt contains about 77 micrograms of iodine.

5. **Vegetables:**

While vegetables are not typically high in iodine, some types such as potatoes and spinach contain small amounts of iodine. One medium-sized potato contains about 60 micrograms of iodine, while a half-cup of cooked spinach can contain up to 15 micrograms of iodine.

6. **Bread:**

Some types of bread are made with iodized salt and can be a good source of iodine. One slice of bread can contain up to 12 micrograms of iodine.

7. **Fruits:**

Fruits such as strawberries and cranberries contain small amounts of iodine. One medium strawberry contains about 3 micrograms of iodine, while a half-cup of cranberries can contain up to 400 micrograms of iodine.

By incorporating these iodine-rich foods into your diet, you can ensure that you're getting enough of this important nutrient.

# How Diet can play a role in getting enough Iodine

Diet plays a crucial role in ensuring that you get enough iodine. Consuming a balanced diet that includes iodine-rich foods is the best way to ensure you meet your daily iodine requirements. Here are some ways that diet can play a role in getting enough iodine:

- **Consume Iodine-Rich Foods**

Iodine can be found in a variety of foods, but one of the finest sources is seafood, specifically seaweed. Kelp, wakame, and nori are just a few examples of the many types of seaweed that can contain up to 2,000 micrograms of iodine per gram. Seaweed is a fantastic source of iodine, and a great way to get more of it into your diet is to eat it on a regular basis or to use it as a flavoring in foods like soups, stews, and salads.

Iodine can also be found in abundance in other forms of seafood, such as shrimp, tuna, and cod, amongst others. For instance, a serving of shrimp that is three ounces contains approximately 23 micrograms of iodine, whereas a serving of cod that is three ounces can have as much as 99 micrograms of iodine. If you want to make sure you get enough iodine in your diet every day, eating a wide variety of seafood is a good way to do so.

However, it is essential to keep in mind that certain types of seafood may also contain high levels of mercury, which, if taken in large quantities, may result in adverse health effects. As a result, it is imperative to pick foods that contain low amounts of mercury and to consume seafood in moderation.

Because of the potential for mercury exposure, pregnant women and children under the age of six should exercise extra caution when consuming large quantities of seafood.

- **Choose Iodized Salt**

Iodized salt is a type of table salt that has been supplemented with iodine. Because of this, using iodized salt is a simple and hassle-free approach to boosting the amount of iodine in your diet. Iodine can be obtained from as little as 77 micrograms of iodized salt in just one gram of this type of salt.

If you want to make sure you get enough iodine in your diet, one easy method to do so is to cook and season your food using iodized salt. It is vital to use iodized salt in moderation since an excessive intake of salt can lead to high blood pressure and other health problems; nevertheless, it is important to note that an excessive intake of salt can lead to high blood pressure and other health problems.

You have the option of consuming other sources of iodine in addition to utilizing iodized salt. Some examples of these other sources are seafood and dairy products. If you want to satisfy your daily iodine requirements without having to rely entirely on iodized salt, including a variety of foods that are rich in iodine in your diet can help you reach those requirements.

If you have certain dietary needs or restrictions, you should consult with a healthcare physician or a trained dietitian in order to receive individualized information on how to fulfill your iodine requirements.

- **Consume a Balanced Diet**

Consuming an appropriate amount of iodine each day is possible if you maintain a healthy, well-rounded diet that features a wide variety of nutrient-dense foods. Although seafood, eggs, and dairy products are all excellent sources of iodine, it is equally important to have a diet that is rich in fruits, vegetables, whole grains, and sources of lean protein.

There is a possibility that some fruits and vegetables, particularly those that were grown in soil that was high in iodine, contain trace levels of iodine. For instance, one potato that is about the size of a medium carries about 60 micrograms of iodine, whereas a half cup of cooked spinach might have as much as 15 micrograms of iodine.

If they are prepared with iodized salt, whole grains such as bread and pasta can also be considered to be valuable sources of iodine. If you choose alternatives that contain whole grains, you may also receive more fiber and other nutrients.

The best method to make sure you are getting enough iodine in your diet on a daily basis is to make sure you are eating a healthy, well-rounded diet that contains a wide variety of foods that are high in nutrients. Consult with a healthcare physician or a qualified dietitian for individualized advice if you have particular dietary requirements or limits.

- **Avoid Excessive Intake of Goitrogens**

Goitrogens are compounds that can be present in certain meals and are known to impede the function of the thyroid as well as the absorption of iodine. Goitrogens can be found in foods like soy products, vegetables from the cruciferous vegetable family including broccoli and cauliflower, and sweet potatoes.

In spite of the fact that these meals are, for the most part, healthful and nutritious, it is essential to eat them in moderation. Iodine deficiency and other health issues can be caused by eating an unhealthy amount of goitrogenic foods, which can result in a reduction in the amount of iodine that is absorbed by the thyroid as well as decreased thyroid function.

It is essential to keep in mind that the goitrogenic effect of certain foods can be mitigated by heating them. For instance, cooking cruciferous vegetables for at least half an hour can lessen the goitrogenic potential of these plants. In addition, eating meals high in iodine in conjunction with foods that cause goiter can assist to counteract any adverse effects on thyroid function.

If you are aware that you have a thyroid problem or an iodine shortage, you should consult with a healthcare professional or a certified dietitian in order to receive individualized advice on how to control the number of goitrogenic foods you consume in your diet.

Consuming a varied diet that includes iodine-rich foods and choosing iodized salt can help ensure you meet your daily iodine requirements. If you suspect you have an iodine deficiency, speak with your healthcare provider for appropriate testing and guidance on iodine supplementation.

# Conclusion

Congratulations, you've reached the end of this beginner's guide on iodine! By now, you should have a good understanding of what iodine is, why it's important, and how to incorporate more of it into your diet. But before you go, let's review some key takeaways and provide some parting words of encouragement.

Firstly, it's crucial to remember that iodine is an essential nutrient that plays a vital role in thyroid function and overall health. Without adequate iodine intake, you may be at risk for a range of health problems, including hypothyroidism, goiter, and cognitive impairments. Therefore, it's essential to assess your iodine intake and make changes to your diet as needed.

Fortunately, there are numerous ways to incorporate more iodine into your diet. Some of the best sources of iodine include seafood, seaweed, eggs, and dairy products. You can also use iodized salt in your cooking or take iodine supplements if recommended by a healthcare provider. By making these simple changes to your diet, you can help support your overall health and well-being.

Despite the many benefits of iodine, it's important to remember that excessive intake can be harmful. Therefore, it's important to speak with a healthcare provider before taking iodine supplements, particularly if you're pregnant or have a history of thyroid problems. By working with a healthcare provider, you can ensure that you're getting adequate levels of iodine without experiencing negative health effects.

In conclusion, incorporating more iodine into your diet can have numerous benefits for your health and well-being. From supporting thyroid function and healthy brain development to boosting the immune system and reducing the risk of certain cancers, iodine is a vital nutrient that shouldn't be overlooked. So why not challenge yourself to incorporate more iodine-rich foods into your diet today? Your body and mind will thank you for it!

# FAQ

**1. Why is iodine important for my health?**

Iodine is a vital nutrient that plays a crucial role in thyroid function and overall health. Without adequate iodine intake, you may be at risk for a range of health problems, including hypothyroidism, goiter, and cognitive impairments.

**2. What are some good food sources of iodine?**

Some of the best sources of iodine include seafood, seaweed, eggs, and dairy products. You can also use iodized salt in your cooking or take iodine supplements if recommended by a healthcare provider.

**3. How much iodine do I need each day?**

The recommended daily intake of iodine varies depending on your age and sex. The World Health Organization recommends that adults consume 150 micrograms of iodine per day, while pregnant and breastfeeding women require higher levels.

**4. Can I get too much iodine?**

Yes, excessive iodine intake can be harmful, particularly in vulnerable populations such as pregnant women or people with thyroid problems. It's important to speak with a healthcare provider before taking iodine supplements to ensure that you're getting adequate levels without experiencing negative health effects.

## 5.  What are the signs of iodine deficiency?

Signs of iodine deficiency may include an enlarged thyroid gland (goiter), fatigue, weight gain, hair loss, and dry skin. Severe cases of iodine deficiency can lead to intellectual disabilities and developmental problems.

## 6.  Are there any risks associated with taking iodine supplements?

While iodine supplements can be beneficial in certain cases, they can also have side effects and interact with certain medications. It's important to speak with a healthcare provider before taking iodine supplements to ensure that they're safe and effective for you.

## 7.  Do I need to worry about iodine deficiency if I live in a developed country?

While iodine deficiency is less common in developed countries, it can still occur, particularly in populations with limited access to iodine-rich foods or iodized salt. It's important to assess your iodine intake and speak with a healthcare provider if you have concerns about your iodine status.

# Resources and Helpful Links

Melse-Boonstra, A., Gowachirapant, S., Jaiswal, N., Winichagoon, P., Srinivasan, K., & Zimmermann, M. B. (2012). Iodine supplementation in pregnancy and its effect on child cognition. Journal of Trace Elements in Medicine and Biology, 26(2–3), 134–136. https://doi.org/10.1016/j.jtemb.2012.03.005

Iodine and Cancer. (2022). Natural Medicine Journal. https://www.naturalmedicinejournal.com/journal/iodine-and-cancer

Rappaport, J. (2017). Changes in Dietary Iodine Explains Increasing Incidence of Breast Cancer with Distant Involvement in Young Women. Journal of Cancer, 8(2), 174–177. https://doi.org/10.7150/jca.17835

Thyroid Cancer Risk Factors | Risk Factors for Thyroid Cancer. (n.d.). https://www.cancer.org/cancer/types/thyroid-cancer/causes-risks-prevention/risk-

factors.html#:~:text=Follicular%20thyroid%20cancers%20ar
e%20more,table%20salt%20and%20other%20foods.

Summers, H. (2022, October 19). Mineral deficiency exposes 19 million babies a year to brain damage risk. The Guardian. https://www.theguardian.com/global-development/2018/mar/02/lack-of-iodine-exposes-19-million-babies-a-year-to-brain-damage-risk#:~:text=Mineral%20deficiency%20exposes%2019%20million%20babies%20a%20year%20to%20brain%20damage%20risk,-This%20article%20is&text=A%20lack%20of%20iodine%20in,a%20new%20report%20has%20warned.

IODINE: Overview, Uses, Side Effects, Precautions, Interactions, Dosing, and Reviews. (n.d.). https://www.webmd.com/vitamins/ai/ingredientmono-35/iodine

Berkheiser, K. (2023, February 1). 9 Healthy Foods That Are Rich in Iodine. Healthline. https://www.healthline.com/nutrition/iodine-rich-foods